Table of Contents

Introduction

LPR Diet also known as Silent reflux is simply a diet for people with Laryngopharyngeal Reflux. This is a diet that opts for natural food choices and avoiding more acidic foods and drinks. Foods that should be avoided are fatty foods, processed foods, chocolate, spicy food, soft drinks and more. LPR occurs when stomach acid enters the esophagus and travels up to the larynx.

LPR stands for laryngopharyngeal reflux. The term reflux describes the backward or return flow of stomach acid. Reflux is often associated with heartburn, the result of stomach acid irritating the throat.

In LPR, stomach acid flows not only back up to the esophagus (food pipe) but also further up to the throat. The problem is that LPR causes unspecific symptoms besides those normally associated with reflux. People often don't realize that their symptoms are caused by LPR, and it can take many years before the condition gets diagnosed. For this reason, LPR is also known as silent reflux.

The silent reflux diet is an alternative treatment that can provide relief from reflux symptoms through simply dietary changes. This diet is a lifestyle change that eliminates or limits trigger foods known to irritate your throat or weaken your esophageal muscles.

Unlike acid reflux or GERD, silent reflux (laryngopharyngeal reflux) can cause little or no symptoms until it has progressed to later stages.

A diet for laryngopharyngeal reflux (LPR) should meet three criteria: The food should be low in acid and fat, and at the same time, improve digestion. You may have likely heard before that diet is the best way to help LPR Symptoms and is one of the most important LPR remedies. This can be effective from 2 different angles. The 2 angles are of course primarily avoiding foods that cause LPR and the worst trigger foods for LPR and acid reflux in general.

The other angle is foods that are soothing to acid reflux, these foods are usually low acid or even alkaline and generally cooling. To give you a few ideas of these foods I would advise you to continue reading.

Chapter One

What is the main cause of LPR?

For gastric juices to travel from your stomach all the way up through your esophagus and into your throat, they have to get past two important guards. These are your upper and lower esophageal sphincters — the muscular valves that seal off your esophagus at the top and bottom. The lower one separates your esophagus and stomach, while the upper one separates your esophagus and throat.

Normal acid reflux happens when something weakens your lower esophageal sphincter (LES), allowing stomach juices to flow back up into your esophagus. LPR happens when your upper esophageal sphincter (UES) also relaxes inappropriately. This allows reflux that's already in your esophagus to creep up higher into your throat. Different things can affect these two sphincters and cause them to relax.

What are some specific causes that can lead to laryngopharyngeal reflux?

A lot of things can affect how well your esophageal sphincters close to keep substances out. Some of these factors weaken the muscles gradually over time, while other factors can affect them temporarily. Most people have more than one factor affecting them. Healthcare providers don't always know exactly which ones caused

LPR, but they often find that if you reduce these factors, your reflux reduces.

1. Breaching your LES

Your lower esophageal sphincter (LES) is the first guard against acid reflux from your stomach into your esophagus. Frequent, substantial acid reflux will cause symptoms of GERD, but you can have a small amount of reflux in your esophagus without feeling it. Your esophagus has many layers of protection against acid reflux, so it takes a lot to wear it down. Your throat doesn't have the same protection.

Common factors that may weaken your LES temporarily include:

Medications: Certain medications can have a relaxing effect on your LES, including:

• Benzodiazepines: a type of sedative.

• Calcium channel blockers: which treat high blood pressure.

• Tricyclic antidepressants: which treat depression and pain.

• NSAIDs (nonsteroidal anti-inflammatory drugs) like aspirin and ibuprofen.

• Theophylline: a common asthma medication.

• Hormone therapy (HT) medications for menopause.

Foods and drinks: Foods and drinks that may have a relaxing effect on your LES include:

• Coffee.

• Chocolate.

• Alcohol.

• Mint.

• Garlic.

• Onions.

Lifestyle habits: Simple things can temporarily weaken your LES by increasing abdominal pressure against it, or by taking away the advantage of gravity, which helps keep it closed.

Lying down or reclining too soon after eating: Sleeping on your back, which submerges your LES inside your stomach contents.

Eating larger meals: which expands your abdomen and increases digestion time.

Wearing tight clothes or belts around your abdomen, especially when sitting.

Common factors that may weaken your LES progressively over time include:

Hiatal hernia: When your stomach bulges up through a hole in your diaphragm, your LES also moves above your diaphragm and loses some of its muscle support system.

Pregnancy: Lots of people get temporary acid reflux during pregnancy when abdominal pressure pushes against your diaphragm and LES. Hormones also contribute.

Obesity: Obesity is another cause of constant abdominal pressure that can weaken your LES over time. It can also affect your hormone levels.

• Smoking: Tobacco smoke has a relaxing effect on your LES. It's also associated with coughing, which can put chronic pressure on your LES. It's a common cause of hiatal hernia.

2. Breaching your UES

Once stomach juices are in your esophagus, it's up to your upper esophageal sphincter (UES) to keep them out of your throat. You may only have a small, unnoticeable amount of reflux in your esophagus, but it doesn't take much to irritate your throat tissues. They don't have the same protective lining as your esophagus, and they also don't have the same mechanisms that wash reflux out, so it stays longer.

Common factors that may weaken or relax your UES include:

• Lying down. Some people have LPR during the night because their esophageal sphincters both relax a little when they lie down.

• Burping. Burping is one reflex that can trigger both your LES and your UES to open. Gas bubbles can carry small amounts of stomach juices into your throat.

• Bending over, exercising or singing. These activities build pressure under your UES, which may weaken it.

• Smoking and alcohol use. These substances have a relaxing effect on both of your esophageal sphincter muscles.

Symptoms: How to Recognize LPR

Because LPR reaches not only the food pipe but also the throat, it causes unspecific symptoms rather than heartburn. These symptoms are caused by inflammation of the mucous membranes in the throat.

The most common symptoms include:

• hoarseness and trouble with speaking

• sore throat

• the feeling of a lump in the throat

• difficulty with swallowing

• excessive mucus in the throat and respiratory tract

• chronic cough

• frequent throat-clearing

• asthma and breathing difficulties

• frequent eructation (burping)

• general irritation of the mucous membranes

• nausea

• enamel erosion and caries

• ear infections

• recurrent flu-like infections

• worsening of other respiratory conditions.

Symptoms in children and infants

The symptoms of silent reflux in infants and children include:

• coughing

• vomiting

• failure to grow and gain weight

• asthma

• a sore throat

• hoarseness

• noisy breathing

• ear infections

• feeding difficulties

• turning blue

• aspiration, or inhaling food and other particles into the lungs

It is common for infants to spit up, but problems with breathing and feeding could be signs of a more serious health problem. A doctor should investigate these symptoms.

In infants and children, LPR can cause:

• Narrowing of the area below the vocal cords

• Contact ulcers

• Recurrent ear infections from problems with eustachian tube function

• Lasting buildup of middle ear fluid

In adults, silent reflux can scar the throat and voice box. It can also increase risk for cancer in the area, affect the lungs, and may irritate conditions such as asthma, emphysema, or bronchitis.

Differences between LPR and GERD

GERD, or gastroesophageal reflux disease, occurs when stomach acid and enzymes backflow into the oesophagus, causing heartburn (burning sensation in the chest) and damage to the esophageal lining. LPR occurs when stomach acid and/or food enzymes backflow all the way back into the lower part of the throat (laryngopharynx). Not everyone who has reflux has LPR.

LPR in the absence of GERD

Many people with LPR do not have symptoms of heartburn. Compared to the esophagus, the voice box and the back of the throat are significantly more sensitive to the effects of acid/pepsin on the surrounding tissues. Acid that passes quickly through the food pipe does not have a chance to irritate the area for too long, However, acid that pools in the throat around the voice box causes prolonged irritation, resulting in the symptoms of LPR.

Throat-clearing alternatives

If you sense a build-up of secretions in the throat, try swallowing or taking a sip of water. You can also use a "silent cough" by pushing as much air as you can from the lungs in a short blast. The only sound should be a rush of air, then swallow.

The Best LPR Diet Is Personalized

What and how you eat can make a huge difference when it comes to managing laryngopharyngeal reflux.

Certain kinds of foods have been shown to contribute to LPR development, trigger symptoms, or both. Dietary changes have been found to improve the condition.

Finding an ideal LPR diet plan for you involves removing common reflux triggers as well as identifying and eliminating your personal trigger foods. Paying attention to when you eat and supporting your gut with probiotics may also be helpful alongside your diet changes.

Foods to avoid

If you decide to pursue the silent reflux diet, doctors recommend eliminating high-fat foods, sweets, and acidic beverages.

Some foods to avoid include:

• whole-fat dairy products

• fried foods

• fatty cuts of meat

• caffeine

• alcohol

• sodas

• onions

• kiwi

• oranges

• limes

• lemons

• grapefruit

• pineapples

• tomatoes and tomato-based foods

It's also important to avoid chocolate, mints, and spicy foods because they're known to weaken the esophageal sphincter. However, each trigger food can affect people differently. Pay close attention to what foods cause you more discomfort or worsen your upper endoscopy results.

Foods to eat

The silent reflux diet is similar to other balanced diets that are usually high in fiber, lean proteins, and vegetables. A 2004 study showed that increasing fiber and limiting salt in your diet can protect against reflux symptoms.

Some of these foods include:

• lean meats

• whole grains wholegrain pasta, wholegrain bread, wholegrain wheat flour

• Condiments: Celtic salt, olive and coconut oil, soybean concentrate, vanilla extract, pea protein, white miso paste

• Raw fruit: Banana, papaya, cantaloupe, honeydew melon, watermelon, lychee and avocado

• apples

• caffeine-free beverages

• water

• leafy green vegetables: Spinach, cos lettuce, rocket, curly kale, bok choy, broccoli, asparagus, celery, cucumbers, courgette, aubergine, potato, sweet potato, carrots(not baby ones), beetroot, chestnut mushrooms, basil, coriander, parsley, rosemary, dried thyme and sage

• legumes

• Dried fruit: Dates, raisins, desiccated coconut

• Nuts and seeds: Cashews, pecans, pistachios, walnuts, pumpkin seeds, sesame seeds, almonds, pine nuts

• Spreads: Fresh, organic peanut and almond butters

• Cheese: Parmesan, mozzarella, other hard cheese

Can you treat LPR naturally?

Some people can solve their LPR with lifestyle adjustments alone. In general, LPR is more likely than GERD to improve without medication, because LPR may be caused by only a small amount of reflux. It takes time for LPR to heal, though, so it may be several months before you can tell if your adjustments are working. Medications called proton pump inhibitors (PPIs) can help speed up the healing process.

What diet and lifestyle changes help with LPR?

Healthcare providers suggest that you:

Eat smaller meals. Try five to six mini meals instead of three bigger ones.

Avoid rich, spicy and acidic foods. These can increase the acid and other irritants in your reflux.

Eat dinner earlier. Try not to recline or lie down for three hours after eating.

Sleep on your left side: This positions your lower esophageal sphincter in an air pocket above your stomach contents, which reduces reflux while you sleep.

Avoid excessive burping: Avoid carbonated beverages and eat slowly so you don't swallow air. If you have chronic burping, you might have a digestive disorder that needs treating.

Reduce abdominal pressure: Wearing loose clothes around your waistline is a start. Reducing abdominal volume is better. A healthcare provider can discuss weight loss options with you.

Quit smoking: Ask your healthcare provider about resources to help you quit.

Reduce alcohol. Talk to your healthcare provider if you think you have alcohol use disorder.

Tips for children

Most infants outgrow silent reflux by their first birthday. Some, however, might need treatment.

Tips that can help include:

feeding the infant smaller, more regular meals

keeping the infant in an upright position for at least 30 minutes when feeding

closely monitoring for signs of breathing or feeding trouble

If breathing or feeding problems develop, seek medical help.

Diet

You may have likely heard before that diet is the best way to help LPR Symptoms and is one of the most important LPR remedies. This can be effective from 2 different angles. The 2 angles are of course primarily avoiding foods that cause LPR and the worst trigger foods for LPR and acid reflux in general.

The other angle is foods that are soothing to acid reflux, these foods are usually low acid or even alkaline and generally cooling. To give you a few ideas of these foods I would recommend watermelon, celery or the likes of cucumber.

All of these are low acidity and are brilliant if you are having a flare up, they have both the cooling effect and the ability to neutralise acid, both of which should help ease and calm symptoms.

Tea

One of the best options to give quick and effective relief is tea. But be careful not any tea will do. There are a couple of teas that I recommend.

The first tea I recommend is chamomile tea, the reason it is great is because it has anti-inflammatory properties which can be soothing for your throat and whole digestive tract.

The other tea I recommend is marshmallow root tea, this tea is brilliant at lining the throat and the whole way down and into the esophagus and stomach, overall in terms of soothing properties this tea is probably your best choice. Here Is the varieties of the teas I recommend on Amazon – chamomile tea & marshmallow root tea.

One thing I recommend when drinking tea is to let it cool down a little before drinking it. Hot water can actually cause the throat more irritation so ideally it's best to let the tea cool down a little before drinking it.

Alkaline Water

Alkaline water is basically water that has a high pH making it alkaline. There are a couple of main benefits to taking this kind of water for someone with LPR. The main cause of throat problems for someone with LPR is because of a digestive enzyme called pepsin coming up from the stomach and into the throat.

The important thing to note with alkaline water is that it deactivates the pepsin. So, if you have any pepsin in your throat causing symptoms drinking this water should deactivate any pepsin that may be in your throat.

Also when you drink this water because it's alkaline this lowers the acidity of the stomach which also can help stop acid reflux and can be generally soothing to the whole digestive tract. For more information on the different kinds of alkaline water and how you can even make your own check this article – Alkaline Water for LPR.

Slippery Elm

Similar to the teas I mentioned above slippery elm can be mixed into water and drank as a tea. It has similar properties like the teas I mentioned earlier. It can be very soothing to a sore throat and generally the larynx.

Slippery elm can also come in the form of lozenges but keep in mind some lozenges have ingredients which can irritate LPR so ideally it's best to just opt for the tea instead.

DGL Licorice

DGL licorice could potentially be helpful for both reflux and the throat and the digestive tract. It may increase the production of mucus which in turn can help ease and soothe the throat and esophagus etc.

Chewable tablets are the best here because it coats everything on the way down into the stomach. Ideally when you are choosing these tablets you want ones with the least added ingredients as possible.

Baking Soda

Something that is often talked about is baking soda, it is one of the best home remedies for LPR. How you want to use baking soda is by mixing a small amount of it with water and mixing well. What this does is it creates an alkaline mixture which helps lower acidity of the digestive tract and the stomach and should help lessen symptoms.

While not the best long-term solution it can be an effective solution if you need a quick and fast ailment.

A Hierarchical LPR Treatment Strategy

Similar to other gut conditions like IBS or SIBO, LPR may have many possible root causes. In this situation, we recommend using a hierarchical approach.

This means applying foundational diet and lifestyle changes first, continuing therapies that give you improvement, and only then moving toward more specific and targeted therapies.

In simplest terms, a hierarchical approach to LPR treatment includes these steps:

1. Modify your diet and eating habits to remove reflux triggers.

2. Improve your gut microbiome with probiotics. Address gut infections with antimicrobials if necessary.

3. Support your stomach acid with betaine HCL if needed.

4. Add additional therapies only if the first three don't provide relief.

Low-acid diet for LPR

Acid activates pepsin, which promotes inflammation. While acidic foods do not cause reflux, they massively exaggerate the symptoms. They add fuel to the fire.

For this reason, people with LPR (or silent reflux) should avoid acidic foods and drinks as far as possible.

There are some misconceptions about which foods are acidic and which are not. The reason for this is the so-called "alkaline diet" trend. In these diets alkaline does not refer to the actual pH of the food. For instance, lemons count as alkaline, even though they have a very low or acidic pH.

Unfortunately, almost all foods and drinks contain some acid. They may not taste sour, but still, they include a small amount of acid. Even bread is mildly acidic.

We cannot eliminate acid because there would be nothing left to eat! The goal of an LPR diet is, therefore, to reduce acid – not to eat a 100% acid-free diet.

Ideally, you should try to abstain from anything with a pH lower than 5 – at least for a while. Once symptoms improve, you can try to reintroduce foods with a pH of as low as 4.

The pH scale is logarithmic. Each number in either direction on the scale corresponds to a 10-fold change in acid content. Foods with a pH of 4 contain 10 times as much acid as foods with a pH of 5 – the acceptable acid content for an anti-reflux diet. Foods with a pH of 3 already contain 100 times as much acid (10 times 10).

When avoiding acid, you should pay special attention to drinks:

• Many beverages, such as Coke, soda and fruit juices, are very acidic. Acid is responsible for the fresh taste of these drinks. Without acid, they would merely taste like stale sugared water. The high sugar content masks the acid so that you cannot taste it. The pH of many soft drinks is about 3, which is very acidic.

• As well as drinks, though, acid foods are also dangerous when you have reflux. You should especially avoid yogurt and fruits.

• Anything pickled also has a high acid content. This is because acids, such as vinegar, are used for preservation.

• I want to stress that it is vital to avoid any foods and drinks with a medium-to-high acid content. Even a few exceptions per week, such as a few sips of a Coke, can exaggerate the LPR problems.

Low-fat diet for LPR

Fat slows down the digestion by reducing gastric motility. This does not mean that you should eliminate fat from your diet, as this would be neither healthy nor constructive. You should aim for a fat content of about 10%. A recipe with 10 g fat, 20 g protein, and 70 g carbohydrates would be excellent. The protein content is not critical – you can eat foods that are low or high in protein. With this strategy, you have a lot of variety and can use fat to improve the taste. The balance is essential. One high-fat meal and four fat-free meals are worse than five meals with the same fat content. Occasional high-fat meals can cause acute, severe reflux that you certainly want to avoid, especially when you are just starting and would like to improve your symptoms rapidly.

Smaller snacks with high-fat content are fine on an empty stomach because it is the total amount of fat that matters. A handful of nuts does not cause problems, while a complete meal with the same fat percentage would cause severe reflux. This fat restriction is mostly meant for the initial part of the diet. Just until you feel better. Later you can try reintroducing gradually fatter foods and see how you are doing.

By the way: Some people do well by reducing carbohydrates instead of fat. This seems to be mostly people who suffer from SIBO (small bacterial intestinal overgrowth). In those people, eating carbs can lead to a lot of gas in the intestines when bacteria ferment the carbohydrates. The belly swells up and puts pressure on the stomach, which leads to reflux. If you feel very gassy and bloated after meals rich in carbohydrates, you might be one of those people. However, SIBO only affects a fraction of patients with reflux. That is why I recommend trying a low-fat diet first because it works better for the far majority of people. No matter if you have SIBO or not, it doesn't change the other components of the diet. Just the relevance of fat and carbohydrates.

The 9 Best Foods to Help Improve Digestion

What you eat—or don't—can play a big role in your digestion, and ultimately your overall health.

Did you know that the health of your gut could actually be a window into the rest of your health? In recent years, research has linked what's happening along your digestive tract to a number of health outcomes—from inflammation, autoimmune disorders, and skin conditions to type 2 diabetes and brain health. It's no wonder that gut health has become such a focus in the world of wellness. Add these 9 foods to your diet for healthy digestion.

oats

"What I love about oats is that they are a prebiotic food, they are inexpensive and they can be used for a variety of recipes, from your morning bowl of oatmeal to an ingredient in your banana bread".

Sauerkraut

Sauerkraut and other fermented foods contain probiotics, which help replenish the inevitable loss of good bacteria in your gut (whether from stress, certain medications, or even environmental factors). Probiotics have been shown to reduce bloating, gas, and other unwanted digestive symptoms. Just like eating a variety of foods is important to a healthy digestive system, so is getting a variety of strains of probiotics (there are hundreds, if not thousands!).

Analysis showed that sauerkraut contains up to 28 different strains, which is more than you'll find in most other probiotic-rich foods or any supplement. And you don't need a lot of sauerkraut to get benefits; one serving is typically just 2 tablespoons and can be added to anything from sandwiches to grain bowls.

Pineapple

"Pineapple is not just a delicious fruit to be enjoyed, it also may support healthy digestion because of the digestive enzyme it contains, called bromelain. Bromelain is known for breaking down proteins in the foods we eat, therefore helping ease the digestive process, leaving you less likely to feel gassy and bloated".

Bromelain has also been shown to potentially counteract certain intestinal pathogens, reducing diarrhea and other digestive symptoms for some.

Chia Seeds

These tiny seeds are an incredible source of fiber. Just 1 ounce (about 2 tablespoons) contains 11 grams of fiber, which is more than one-third of the daily recommended amount. It's the soluble fiber that actually helps them make a pudding-like texture when soaked in a liquid, and this same fiber helps absorb water in your gut.

"This type of fiber not only helps promote and support beneficial bacteria in your gut, but it can also reduce constipation by promoting healthy, regular bowel movements".

Apples

"Apples contain a fiber called pectin, which is very subtle on the gut compared to others like chicory root or inulin which may cause excessive bloating or abdominal discomfort in those with existing digestive conditions".

Pectin has also been shown to provide protective benefits in the lining of the gut—potentially keeping out unwanted pathogens—and may enhance nutrient absorption. All varieties of apples offer similar benefits, so choose the ones you like best.

Beans

Beans, beans, the magical fruit ... you know how the rest goes. But that slightly unpleasant side effect is actually a normal—and positive—response to eating a fiber called oligosaccharides.

The fiber in beans is fermented by the good bacteria in your gut, which keeps them doing their important job of allowing nutrients into your bloodstream and keeping toxins out. "Mixed bean tins are one of my top cupboard staples. In fact one of my top tips for upping your fiber and plant diversity intake is to go for mixed beans with three or four different types, instead of just the kidney beans".

Broccoli

Broccoli, along with other cruciferous vegetables like cabbage, cauliflower, and Brussels sprouts, has been linked to better digestive health and diversity of the microbiota in your gut. Cruciferous vegetables are also known for reducing the risk of colorectal cancer and lowering inflammation of the colon. It's hypothesized that intestinal fermentation of the prebiotic fiber in these vegetables helps form short-chain fatty acids that may reduce inflammation.

This can come with a side of gas, so if you're not regularly eating cruciferous vegetables already, add them to your diet in small amounts to start.

Bananas

Bananas—especially those that are less ripe—contain resistant starch, which can feed the good bacteria in your gut, improving the gut microbiome. As they get riper, the resistant starch turns to sugar, but some beneficial starch remains.

Bananas are such a versatile fruit, so get creative with how you eat them—for breakfast, as a pre-workout snack, or dipped in chocolate or nut butter for dessert.

OK, so we know this isn't technically a food, but we couldn't ignore the importance of hydration when it comes to healthy digestion. "Fluids work to help break down the food you eat so your body can absorb those nutrients to keep you in good health".

Water and fiber work together to help keep you regular. "Fiber pulls the fluid into the colon to help produce softer, bulkier stools that are easier to pass". Sometimes if people increase fiber intake too quickly and don't drink enough water, they can struggle with digestive symptoms as well. So, drink up! Don't love plain water? Try adding in fresh fruit, citrus, or some herbs for a flavor boost.

NOTE

A diverse, plant-rich diet is the best way to support healthy digestion. But adding these specific foods may give your gut a little extra boost. It's also important to remember that "gut health isn't just about what you eat. Sleep, stress, and exercise can each have a big impact too. So, take into account your entire lifestyle and make sure to tackle sleep, stress, and movement, in addition to food, for the best digestive health.

How to cure silent reflux action

Avoid Overeating

Of course, while following these suggested diet steps is essential to recover from LPR there are other elements which should also be followed. One of the most important things to consider is the size of the portions you are eating. When I say this, if you are eating large portions where you feel like you ate too much, or you feel bloated after then this is something for you to think about.

The reason why you don't want to eat large portions is because of the pressure it puts on the lower esophageal sphincter (LES). If you didn't know the LES is the valve above the stomach which is designed to close once foods enter the stomach and then the digestion process starts.

For a lot of people, a LES that is not functioning correctly can be the root cause of their LPR in the first place. When someone eats a bigger meal it puts more pressure on the LES, this higher pressure means more likelihood that the LES will relax and open and thus the acid will reflux up causing you your symptoms in the first place. Not only do you have this effect but because of this overeating it can cause the LES to slowly degrade and degenerate over time. This could be over a period of months/years for most people and for a lot of them could even be how they got LPR initially. You can read more about the importance of the LES and its role in LPR here.

The simple solution in this situation is to eat smaller portion sizes. You shouldn't eat more than what your stomach can hold at one time. For reference this is about the size of your fist. Keep in mind this doesn't mean to eat less throughout the day, but it means to spread it out more evenly between more meals and snacks instead of fewer larger meals.

Luckily if you do this it will not only mean less pressure on the LES and less reflux symptoms but any previous damage that has been done over the past months/years of overeating can be gradually healed over time and will return to normal function!

While it may seem a bit overwhelming at first, making these diet and eating changes can significantly lower your silent reflux symptoms, and even make them vanish for some! And while it may not to be easy to give up some of your favorite foods and beverages, living pain free and lessening the damage to your digestive systems is definitely worth it in the long run!

LPR Treatment Success

Usually for people who follow my advice see good improvement usually within 2 weeks time. For some it can take a little longer but it's just important to remain consistent with it.

Eating habits

As well as a person changing the food they eat, they can also make adjustments to the way they eat and live to reduce silent reflux.

For example, a person with silent reflux may wish to:

• Avoid bending over within 2 hours of eating.

• Eat smaller meals throughout the day instead of three big meals.

• Avoid lying down within 3 hours of eating.

• Avoid eating or drinking anything before going to bed.

• Inserting a 4-inch wedge under the bed to elevate the head when sleeping.

Motility Supports and Prokinetics for Reflux

Some studies suggest that slow gut motility (the movement of food through the digestive tract) may be an underlying cause of reflux . Research suggests this may be true, as blends of prokinetic herbs, like Iberogast or RKT (a Japanese herbal blend including ginger and ginseng), have been shown to improve reflux, heartburn, and lower esophageal sphincter function.

• Supporting your gut motility with such herbal products may improve your LPR symptoms.

• And don't forget the eating behaviors that improve motility as well:

• Avoid snacking between meals.

• Don't eat 2-3 hours before bed.

• Avoid late-night snacking to ensure a long overnight fast. This allows your "migrating motor complex" to perform its daily cleaning cycle on your intestines.

Treatment for laryngopharyngeal reflux begins with addressing the cause. Often, there's no one obvious cause, so healthcare providers focus on diet and lifestyle adjustments to reduce all possible contributing causes. This might mean addressing habits like smoking, drinking alcohol or coffee, or adjusting the way you eat and sleep. Some people might need treatment for an underlying condition, like an esophageal disorder.

Medication

Medication usually plays a limited role in treating laryngopharyngeal reflux. For example, your provider might prescribe proton pump inhibitors for several months while you aim to reduce your reflux with lifestyle changes. These neutralize the acid in your reflux and also coat and protect the tissues in your throat while they heal. If this approach works, you'll be able to discontinue medication after a while.

If you continue to have symptoms, you might need to use an acid-blocking medication or another medication long-term. Acid blockers like proton pump inhibitors and H2 blockers can help when you continue to have reflux despite efforts to reduce it. These medications reduce the acid content in your reflux. Medications called alginates can help protect against other irritants in your reflux, like enzymes.

Your doctor may suggest one or more medications for your condition. Be sure to take them as directed by your doctor. It is important to pay attention to the timing of some medications for LPR. These may work best if taken 30 to 60 minutes before a meal. There are several over-the-counter (OTC) medications your doctor may consider based on your needs, including:

• Histamine blockers that reduce acid production, such as famotidine (Pepcid) and cimetidine (Tagamet)

• Proton pump inhibitors that stop stomach acid from forming, such as rabeprazole (Aciphex), esomeprazole (Nexium), lansoprazole (Prevacid), omeprazole (Prilosec), and pantatoprazole (Protonix)

• Alginates derived from kelp that physically block the reflux of stomach content into the esophagus without having to absorb a medication, such as sodium alginate (Reflux Gourmet), sodium alginate (Gaviscon Advance), and sodium alginate, aloe vera (Esophageal Guardian)

Some of these medications are also available by prescription at a higher dose, which may be more effective if results are not adequate with OTC options.

Finally, certain medications may increase the acid levels in your stomach and aggravate LPR symptoms. It is important to review all your medications with your doctor, including OTC medications and dietary supplements. Do not stop any medications without speaking with the doctor who prescribed them.

What's the outlook with laryngopharyngeal reflux (LPR)?

Getting an accurate diagnosis, discovering the contributing causes and targeting them with the right treatment can be a process. But once the way is clear, treatment for LPR is usually brief and effective. Most people won't need long-term prescription medications or other interventions. The key to recovery lies in making helpful lifestyle changes and taking care to protect your throat and voice while they heal.

Is Water Good for Acid Reflux?

Water can be good but it can depends on the acidity of the water. The higher the pH of the water, the more likely it will be good for your acid reflux. Ideally water with a pH over 7 at least but more ideally over 8 pH will likely be helpful for acid reflux due to it helping neutralise the acid.

Diagnosis and Tests

How can you tell if you have LPR?

If you have chronic hoarseness, there's a 50% chance you have LPR. Look out for other related symptoms, as well. Most people with LPR are unaware of having acid reflux. You might think that you have allergies or an endless cold. Actually, many people develop their first symptoms of LPR shortly after an infection that irritated their throat. This irritation set the stage for reflux to do its own damage.

Most Effective Treatment for LPR

Usually the top 2 things I recommend people do is the strict low acid diet and taking Gaviscon Advance (UK version) 30 minutes after meals and before bedtime.

Management and Treatment

How do I get rid of LPR?

The approach to treating LPR depends on how severe it is and how serious the cause is. In many cases, there's no serious problem with your esophageal sphincter muscles, and diet and lifestyle changes can make a real difference in reducing LPR reflux. Medication can help heal your tissues as these adjustments begin to take effect. But some people do need more extensive treatment than others.

How can I take care of my throat and voice to help them heal?

Healthcare providers suggest that you:

Use your voice gently. Avoid speaking for long periods, like a long phone conversation or formal presentation. Try to minimize shouting, whispering, coughing and clearing your throat.

Stay hydrated. Drink lots of water and avoid drying substances, like caffeine, alcohol and menthol cough drops. Herbal teas with marshmallow or honey can be soothing.

Avoid smoke. Whether it's you or someone around you who's smoking, exposure to smoke will irritate your throat and vocal cords. It also makes reflux worse.

NOTE

Symptoms affecting your throat, vocal cords and sinuses can have many causes. Most are temporary, like infections and allergies. When these symptoms continue for a long time without any obvious cause, it can be frustrating, as well as confusing. Most people don't think of acid reflux as a possible cause of these symptoms, especially when they aren't aware of having it. But that can be the case with LPR.

It only takes a small amount of acid reflux — which includes erosive enzymes like pepsin and stomach acid — to affect your sensitive throat and voice. An even smaller amount may escape through your throat into your respiratory system and do damage there. Fortunately, this also means that small adjustments are often enough to manage it. Treatment for LPR is usually successful and short-term.

What are the complications of LPR?

Laryngopharyngeal reflux may cause:

Excessive mucus and frequent infections:Stomach acid interferes with the normal mechanisms that clear mucus and infections out of your throat and sinuses. Mucus exists to trap infections and help clear them out. When mucus doesn't get cleared out, infections don't, either.

Chronic voice and throat irritation: Chronic voice and throat irritation can interfere with your ability to speak and swallow. Over time, it can cause vocal cord lesions (growths) to develop. Long-term vocal inflammation (laryngitis) is also a risk factor for developing laryngeal cancer.

Respiratory complications: Acid in your larynx may pass through your trachea (windpipe) into your bronchial tubes and lungs. You can inhale tiny acid particles without realizing it, especially in your sleep (silent aspiration). This can cause bronchial inflammation and infections.

How does the LPR diet plan counteract symptoms?

It starts with a 2-week, strict, acid-free diet, a kind of digestive system detox program. It includes no fruit, except bananas and melons, and the main beverage is water – at least 8 cups a day, non-carbonated.

More than half my patients have seen great relief after this period.

Then certain foods can be added back in. I recommend people keep a food diary to see if any of these new items trigger symptoms.

Why Nutrition is Important for a Weight Loss Diet?

What do all diet programs for weight loss have in common? In order to see results you generally need to create a calorie deficit over time. Without a reduction in calories, you may not lose weight.

That being said, reducing calories too much can leave you feeling unsatisfied and restricted. This leads to cravings and the inability to control your food intake when highly palatable foods are in front of you.

Does this sound familiar? You overate tonight so you decide to eat less tomorrow. Another day or two of very low calories go by to make up for overeating a few days ago and you end up binging again - and the cycle continues.

To prevent this, avoid reducing daily calories beyond the 250-500 recommended by healthcare professionals.

7-Day Sample Weight Loss Menu

This one-week meal plan was designed for a person who requires about 2,000 calories per day but aims to achieve weight loss through an intake of 1,500 to 1,750 calories per day with 3 meals and 2 snacks. Your daily calorie goal may vary. Learn what it is below, then make tweaks to the plan to fit your specific needs. Consider working with a registered dietitian or speaking with another healthcare provider to assess and plan for your dietary needs more accurately.

To promote weight loss, this plan is low-carb, high protein, and moderate fat. The macronutrient ratios of this meal plan are 25% carbohydrates, 40% protein, and 35% dietary fat. Food swaps or replacements are fine as long as you do so with similar menu items and portion sizes.

We've researched and reviewed the best weight loss meal delivery services. If you're in the market for a meal delivery service, explore which option may be best for you.

Day 1

Breakfast

• 3 large scrambled eggs

• 1 slice whole wheat toast

• Micronutrients: 350 calories, 21 grams protein, 17 grams carbohydrates, and 21 grams fat

• Snack

• 1 small container (5.3 ounces) plain nonfat Greek Yogurt

• 1/4 cup blueberries

• 1-ounce cashew pieces

• Micronutrients: 272 calories, 20 grams protein, 20 grams carbohydrates, and 14 grams fat

Lunch

- 4 ounces grilled chicken breast

- 2 cups chopped romaine lettuce

- 1/4 cup sliced strawberries

- 2 tablespoons sunflower seeds

- 1 tablespoon olive oil

- 1 tablespoon balsamic vinegar

- Micronutrients: 418 calories, 38 grams protein, 11 grams carbohydrates, and 26 grams fat

Snack

- 1 scoop whey protein powder mixed in 1 cup nonfat milk

- Micronutrients: 193 calories, 28 grams protein, 18 grams carbohydrates, and 1 grams fat

Dinner

- 4 ounces grilled sirloin steak

- 1 small baked potato

- 1 cup steamed mixed vegetables

- Micronutrients: 449 calories, 36 grams protein, 39 grams carbohydrates, and 17 grams fat

Daily Totals: 1,683 calories, 144 grams protein, 106 grams carbohydrates, and 79 grams fat

Note that beverages are not included in this meal plan. Individual fluid needs vary based on age, sex, activity level, and medical history. For optimal hydration, experts generally recommend drinking approximately 9 cups of water per day for women and 13 cups of water per day for men.5 When adding beverages to your meal plan, consider their calorie count. Aim to reduce or eliminate consumption of sugar-sweetened beverages, and opt for water when possible.

Day 2
Breakfast

• 1/3 cup dry oats (cook in water and a dash of salt and cinnamon)

• 4 large scrambled egg whites

• 1 ounce slivered almonds

• Micronutrients: 340 calories, 24 grams protein, 25 grams carbohydrates, and 17 grams fat

Snack

• 1 medium apple

• 2 tablespoons natural peanut butter

• Micronutrients: 316 calories, 9 grams protein, 38 grams carbohydrates, and 17 grams fat

Lunch

• 4 ounces solid white tuna in water (drained)

- 1 tablespoon olive oil mayonnaise

- 16 thin wheat crackers

- Micronutrients: 327 calories, 29 grams protein, 22 grams carbohydrates, and 13 grams fat

Snack

- 1 scoop whey protein powder mixed in coffee or water

- 1-ounce almonds

- Micronutrients: 280 calories, 26 grams protein, 12 grams carbohydrates, and 16 grams fat

Dinner

- 6 ounces grilled chicken breast

- 1 cup steamed broccoli

- Micronutrients: 306 calories, 54 grams protein, 11 grams carbohydrates, and 6 grams fat

Daily Totals: 1,569 calories, 141 grams protein, 108 grams carbohydrates, and 70 grams fat

Day 3
Breakfast

- 6 ounces 2% cottage cheese

- 1/4 cup pineapple chunks

- 1-ounce cashew pieces

• Micronutrients: 337 calories, 22 grams protein, 27 grams carbohydrates, and 17 grams fat

Snack

• 1/2 cup guacamole

• 1 red bell pepper, sliced

• Micronutrients: 213 calories, 3 grams protein, 18 grams carbohydrates, and 17 grams fat

Lunch

• 6 ounces roasted turkey deli meat

• 1 slice provolone cheese

• 1 (6-7 inch) flour tortilla or wrap

• Micronutrients: 340 calories, 43 grams protein, 15 grams carbohydrates, and 12 grams fat

Snack

• 1 cup salted and prepared edamame in the pod

• 1 cup sliced carrots

• Micronutrients: 238 calories, 20 grams protein, 25 grams carbohydrates, and 8 grams fat

Dinner

• 6 ounce 97% lean ground beef burger

• 1 slider-size hamburger bun

• 2 slices tomato

• 2 lettuce leaves

• 1 tablespoon ketchup

• 2 slices red onion

• Micronutrients: 432 calories, 54 grams protein, 25 grams carbohydrates, and 11 grams fat

Daily Totals: 1,559 calories, 143 grams protein, 110 grams carbohydrates, and 65 grams fat

Day 4
Breakfast

• 1 serving Oatmeal Cottage Cheese Waffles

• 1/2 cup raspberries

• Micronutrients: 262 calories, 21 grams protein, 21 grams carbohydrates, and 11 grams fat

Snack

• 2 large hard-boiled eggs

• 1 part-skim mozzarella string cheese

• 1 cup grapes

• 1 cup sliced carrots

Micronutrients: 359 calories, 21 grams protein, 41 grams carbohydrates, and 14 grams fat

Lunch

• 6 ounces grilled chicken breast

• 2 cups romaine lettuce

• 1/4 cup corn kernels

• 1/4 cup black beans

• 1/4 avocado

• 1 tablespoon lime juice

• 1 tablespoon olive oil

• 1 tablespoon chopped cilantro

Micronutrients: 562 calories, 57 grams protein, 26 grams carbohydrates, and 28 grams fat

Snack

• 1 scoop whey protein powder mixed in coffee or water

• Micronutrients: 110 calories, 20 grams protein, 6 grams carbohydrates, and 1 grams fat

Dinner

• 6 ounces 99% fat-free ground turkey breast, sauteed in 1 teaspoon olive oil and mixed with 1/4 cup marinara sauce

• 2 cups steamed zucchini noodles

• Micronutrients: 284 calories, 40 grams protein, 12 grams carbohydrates, and 9 grams fat

Daily Totals: 1,578 calories, 159 grams protein, 107 grams carbohydrates, and 63 grams fat

Day 5
Breakfast

• Smoothie: 1 scoop whey protein powder, 1 small frozen banana, 1 tablespoon peanut butter, 1 cup nonfat milk, ice

• Micronutrients: 383 calories, 34 grams protein, 45 grams carbohydrates, and 10 grams fat

Snack

• 1/4 cup pistachios, in the shell

• Micronutrients: 175 calories, 6.5 grams protein, 8 grams carbohydrates, and 14 grams fat

Lunch

• 4 ounces deli roast beef

• 1 slice provolone cheese

• 1 slice rye bread

• 2 slices red onion

• 2 slices tomato

• Micronutrients: 337 calories, 34 grams protein, 18 grams carbohydrates, and 11 grams fat

Snack

• 1 small container (5.3 ounces) plain nonfat Greek Yogurt

• 1-ounce almonds

• Micronutrients: 258 calories, 21 grams protein, 11 grams carbohydrates, and 15 grams fat

Dinner

• 4 ounces grilled chicken breast

• 1/2 cup cooked brown rice

• 1 tablespoon butter

• 1 cup steamed mixed vegetables

• Micronutrients: 424 calories, 38 grams protein, 33 grams carbohydrates, and 17 grams fat

Daily Totals: 1,578 calories, 133 grams protein, 115 grams carbohydrates, and 68 grams fat

Day 6

Breakfast

Overnight Oats: Combine the following in a bowl, cover and refrigerate overnight. Top with 1 ounce chopped walnuts.

• 1/3 cup dry oatmeal

• 2 ounces plain nonfat Greek yogurt

• 1 scoop whey protein powder

• dash salt

• 1/4 cup nonfat milk

• dash of cinnamon

• Micronutrients: 464 calories, 34 grams protein, 38 grams carbohydrates, and 22 grams fat

Snack

• 1 cup salted and prepared edamame, in the pod

• 1 cup sliced carrots

• Micronutrients: 238 calories, 20 grams protein, 25 grams carbohydrates, and 8 grams fat

Lunch

• Quesadilla: 3 ounces grilled chicken breast, 1/4 cup shredded Mexican cheese, and 1 (6-7 inch) flour tortilla; serve with 2 tablespoons salsa

• Micronutrients: 306 calories, 37 grams protein, 17 grams carbohydrates, and 11 grams fat

Snack

• 6 ounces 2% cottage cheese

• 1 medium peach

• Micronutrients: 196 calories, 19 grams protein, 22 grams carbohydrates, and 4 grams fat

Dinner

• 6 ounces grilled salmon

• 6 large steamed asparagus spears

• Micronutrients: 370 calories, 40 grams protein, 3 grams carbohydrates, and 21 grams fat

Daily Totals: 1,573 calories, 149 grams protein, 107 grams carbohydrates, and 67 grams fat

Day 7

Breakfast

• 4 egg white omelet with 1/4 cup sliced mushrooms, 1 cup spinach, and 1/4 avocado

• 1 slice wheat toast

• Micronutrients: 250 calories, 20 grams protein, 23 grams carbohydrates, and 8 grams fat

Snack

• Smoothie: 2/3 cup plain nonfat Greek Yogurt, 1 cup nonfat milk, 1/4 cup frozen blueberries, 1/4 cup frozen strawberries, 3 tablespoons hemp seeds, 1/2 frozen banana

• Micronutrients: 425 calories, 34 grams protein, 42 grams carbohydrates, and 16 grams fat

Lunch

• 6 ounces grilled salmon

• 6 steamed asparagus spears

• Micronutrients: 370 calories, 40 grams protein, 3 grams carbohydrates, and 21 grams fat

Snack

• 2 hard-boiled eggs

• Micronutrients: 155 calories, 13 grams protein, 1 grams carbohydrates, and 11 grams fat

Dinner

• 4 ounces grilled chicken breast

• 1 cup steamed stir fry vegetables

• 1/2 cup cooked white rice

• 1 tablespoon teriyaki sauce

• Micronutrients: 457 calories, 43 grams protein, 40 grams carbohydrates, and 15 grams fat

Daily Totals: 1,657 calories, 150 grams protein, 110 grams carbohydrates, and 71 grams fat

How to Meal Plan for a Weight Loss Diet

Determine your calorie needs: Start by figuring out how many calories you need to eat per day by using a daily calorie calculator. From there, determine how many grams of protein, carbs, and fats by using macronutrient ratios like the ones shared above. Divide those numbers by the amount of meals and snacks to determine portion sizes.

Write down what you want to eat: Take a few moments to make a list of meals and snacks you'd enjoy eating. Plug those into the week ahead to create a meal plan.

Utilize leftovers: Make an extra portion at dinner so you can have it for lunch the next day. That way you're spending less time cooking.

Don't be afraid to copy and paste days: It's OK to eat the same thing sometimes, in fact, doing so can make your life easier. You know you like the food and there's less thought needed to figure out what you're going to eat.

Stock your fridge and pantry: Shop in advance for the foods you need on your meal plan that way you're always prepared when mealtime comes.

Prep meals the night before whenever possible: Making food the night before can save time in the morning when you're rushing to get out the door. And when you come home from a long day of work, the last thing you want to do is cook. Having dinner already prepped makes it easy to heat up when it's time to eat.

How Do You Treat LPR Naturally?

The best way to treat LPR naturally is through a strict low acid diet plan like the Wipeout Diet where you avoid foods and drinks with a pH of under 5 – a good starting point – LPR Diet Advice. There are also other things that can help, for example not eating within 3 hours before bedtime and also not eating a lot in one sitting.

Can You Cure Silent Reflux?

Yes in most cases silent reflux can be cured or at least vastly improved. The best way is through a low acid diet and some lifestyle changes.

How Long Does LPR Take To Heal?

For every person it can be different. For some people simply eliminating trigger foods will be enough to completely resolve problems. Whereas for others they will have to stick to a strict low acid diet to see good improvements but not complete resolvement.

Is Honey Good for Reflux?

Generally I recommend people with LPR avoid honey when starting the diet because it tends to be a little too acidic. Manuka honey is usually more alkaline than regular honey so if you are to take honey it's best to take manuka. After you start to feel better you can start to take honey more regularly without being concerned.

Chapter Two

Diet for acid reflux

There are several potential ways to include generally healthy foods in small meals throughout the day.

Breakfast

• For breakfast, a person may wish to consider eating oatmeal or another wholegrain cereal. Wholegrain cereals can be filling, which means that a person will need less to feel full until lunch.

• People can add non-citric fruits such as coconut flakes to their oatmeal for added flavor.

Lunch

For lunch, a person may wish to consider a grilled chicken breast salad. The grilled chicken breast provides lean protein that can be filling.

Snacks

• Eating snacks can help a person feel full throughout the day. A person can incorporate these to ensure that they are eating smaller meals throughout the day instead of only three larger meals.

• A person could eat one hard-boiled egg or a piece of nonacidic fruit, such as melon.

• Crackers and hummus may also satisfy hunger without causing additional stomach acid to form.

Dinner

• A person could eat a grilled fish fillet with steamed vegetables, such as broccoli, for a filling meal that should not aggravate silent reflux.

• When planning dinners, a person should try to include a variety of healthy foods, such as protein sources, whole grains, vegetables, and fruits.

Dessert

For dessert, a person can choose foods such as:

• fruit ices

• nonacidic fruits

• gelatin products

Other at-home remedies

According to medical professionals, a person with silent reflux can also try:

• not smoking or using tobacco

• not wearing clothing that is too tight

- lying on the left side instead of the right

- chewing gum containing bicarbonate of soda

- maintaining a moderate weight

- taking any prescribed medication as a doctor instructs

Breakfast meal plan idea for LPR Diet

Starting your day with a healthy and LPR-friendly breakfast is essential for maintaining a balanced diet. Here are two delicious recipes that will not only satisfy your taste buds but also support your acid reflux management.

Recipe 1: LPR-friendly Smoothie

A smoothie is a great way to kickstart your morning with a refreshing and nutrient-packed drink. This LPR-friendly smoothie recipe combines a variety of ingredients to create a delicious and soothing blend.

To make the smoothie, gather the following ingredients:

1 ripe banana

1 cup of almond milk

1 tablespoon of almond butter

1 tablespoon of honey

1/2 cup of spinach

Blend all the ingredients together until you achieve a smooth and creamy consistency. The ripe banana adds natural sweetness while the almond milk and butter provide a creamy texture. The spinach adds a dose of vitamins and minerals, making this smoothie a nutritious choice.

Enjoy this smoothie as a light and satisfying breakfast option. Its gentle and soothing properties make it an excellent choice for those with LPR.

Recipe 2: Oatmeal with banana (LPR-friendly Toppings)

Oatmeal is a classic breakfast choice that can be easily adapted to suit your LPR diet. This recipe combines the comforting warmth of oatmeal with LPR-friendly toppings that enhance both taste and nutrition.

To prepare this oatmeal recipe, follow these simple steps:

Cook 1/2 cup of steel-cut or rolled oats according to package instructions.

Once cooked, transfer the oatmeal to a bowl.

Add sliced bananas on top for a natural sweetness.

Sprinkle a dash of ground cinnamon for added flavor.

Drizzle a small amount of honey to enhance the taste.

This oatmeal recipe provides a hearty and nourishing start to your day. The combination of oats, bananas, cinnamon, and honey creates a delicious flavor profile that will keep you satisfied until your next meal.

Remember, maintaining a healthy and LPR-friendly breakfast routine is crucial for managing acid reflux symptoms. These recipes offer a variety of flavors and textures while still aligning with your dietary needs. Start your day off right with these nutritious and delicious breakfast options!

Recipe 1: Grilled Chicken Salad

For a satisfying midday meal, try this grilled chicken salad:

Grill a boneless, skinless chicken breast and slice it into thin strips.

Combine your choice of mixed greens, cherry tomatoes, cucumber slices, and shredded carrots.

Drizzle with extra virgin olive oil and a squeeze of fresh lemon.

This refreshing salad is packed with flavor and essential nutrients, without triggering LPR symptoms.

Recipe 2: Quinoa and Vegetable Stir-fry

Whip up a quick and delicious stir-fry packed with protein and veggies:

Cook 1 cup of quinoa according to package instructions.

Sauté a mix of colorful vegetables, such as bell peppers, broccoli, and snap peas, in a non-stick pan.

Add cooked quinoa and stir-fry sauce of your choice, and cook until heated through.

This nutritious and flavorful meal will keep you satiated while supporting your LPR diet efforts.

Dinner meal plan idea for LPR Diet

Enjoy a heart-healthy and LPR-friendly dinner with this simple recipe:

Recipe 1: Baked Salmon with Steamed Vegetables

Preheat the oven to 400°F (200°C).

Season a salmon fillet with salt, pepper, and your choice of herbs.

Place the salmon on a baking sheet lined with parchment paper and bake for 12-15 minutes, or until cooked through.

Steam your favorite vegetables, such as broccoli, carrots, and asparagus, until tender.

The baked salmon and steamed vegetables provide a satisfying and nourishing meal that won't exacerbate LPR symptoms.

Recipe 2: Whole Grain Pasta with Tomato-Free Sauce

Satisfy your pasta cravings with this LPR-friendly recipe:

Cook your preferred whole grain pasta according to package instructions.

In a separate pan, sauté minced garlic in olive oil.

Add a can of pureed butternut squash and a splash of vegetable broth. Simmer until heated through.

Toss the cooked pasta in the sauce, and season with salt, pepper, and dried herbs of your choice.

This tomato-free pasta dish provides a delicious alternative while keeping LPR symptoms at bay.

Here are some LPR diet recipes :

Jordan's Quickie Poached Salmon with Rosemary
4 servings

Ingredients

• 4 salmon filets (4 oz. each)

• 4 sprigs fresh rosemary

• 4 half-slices fresh lemon

• 1 teaspoon olive oil

Preparation

1. Place each filet skin-side down on a sheet of aluminum foil large enough to wrap entire filet.

2. Place lemon and rosemary on the filet and drizzle ¼ tsp of the olive oil. Season with salt as needed.

3. Wrap each filet in foil and place in a baking pan in the oven at 350°F for 10-15 minutes.

4. To serve: Remove from oven, unwrap foil, remove the lemon (do not squeeze it on the filet) and the rosemary.

5. Serve with rice and your favorite steamed greens.

Notes: Prep time is about 5 minutes for the salmon. The tightly wrapped foil allows the filets to steam. The rosemary (or other herbs of your choice) and the slice of lemon impart great flavor.

Since you're not squeezing the lemon on the fish, you can avoid its acidity while enjoying the flavor – especially from the lemon skin that steams along with the filets.

You can leave out the olive oil drizzle if you prefer.

For accompanying vegetables, steam asparagus, broccoli or spinach.

Nutritional Facts

Per serving:

514 calories

38g protein

82g carbohydrates

4g fat

Sweet Potato and Green Bean Salad

Serves 6

Ingredients

• 1 lb. green beans (both ends removed, cut into pieces about 2 inches long)

• 1 lb. sweet potatoes (peeled and cut into 1-inch cubes)

• 1 cup pineapple juice

• 1/4 cup maple syrup

• 2 tablespoons olive oil

• Zest from 1 lemon (washed, to yield about 2 tsp)

• 1/4 teaspoon ground cumin

• 2 bay leaves

• 2 tablespoons soy sauce

• 1 teaspoon sesame seeds

• 3 cups baby arugula or watercress

Preparation

1. Place the green beans in boiling salted water and cook until al dente. Remove and place in ice-cold water. Drain.

2. Place the pineapple juice, cumin and bay leaves in a small saucepan. Simmer on low heat and reduce by half.

3. In a bowl, mix the maple syrup, pineapple juice reduction, and soy sauce.

4. Place the olive oil in a pan over high heat, add the sweet potatoes, and cook until golden brown on all sides.

5. Place the sweet potatoes in a bowl and add the green beans, lemon zest, and the maple and pineapple dressing. Toss until mixed.

6. Place the arugula (or watercress) on the bottom of a plate and the vegetables on top. Sprinkle with the toasted sesame seeds.

7. Serve immediately.

Notes: It is important to chill the green beans in ice-cold water immediately after cooking or they will lose their bright green color.

Mixing the dressing with the sweet potatoes while they are still warm allows even distribution of the dressing throughout the salad.

The salad should be served at room temperature. If potatoes are too warm, the watercress will wilt.

Nutrition Facts

Per serving:

253 calories

3g protein

39g carbohydrates

10g fat

OMG (Oh My God) Banana Oatmeal Pancakes
Serves 4

Ingredients

• 2 tablespoons light-brown sugar

• 1/2 cup oat flour

• 1/2 cup all-purpose flour

• 1 teaspoon baking powder

• 1/2 teaspoon salt

• 1/8 teaspoon nutmeg

• 2 large eggs

• 3 bananas, blended or food-processed

• 2 tablespoons (1 oz.) nonfat sour cream or buttermilk

• Milk (to consistency)

• 1 tablespoon butter (for cooking)

• Maple syrup, as desired

Preparation

1. Mix light-brown sugar, oat flour, all-purpose flour, baking powder, salt and nutmeg together in a bowl.

2. Whisk in sour cream or buttermilk, eggs and bananas.

3. If the mixture is too thick, add milk a few tablespoons at a time.

4. Preheat a nonstick pan over low to medium heat. Wipe a paper towel that has been rubbed with butter on the

pan's bottom. (Remove excess butter with the same paper towel and use again before cooking next pancake.)

5. With a ladle, pour some batter into the pan.

6. Flip pancake when underside is golden brown; cook until no longer wet inside.

7. Keep all pancakes warm until ready.

8. Serve with maple syrup; can be topped with diced apples.

Notes: use Canadian D-grade maple syrup (equivalent of grade C in the U.S.) for its darker color and stronger flavor.

• Cooking in a non-stick pan allows you to use butter sparingly.

• You can make your own oat flour by blending rolled oats in a food processor or blender until fine.

• If you make the batter the night before, don't add the baking powder until just before cooking. This batter will be slightly darker, but the result will be just as delicious.

• Adding a tiny bit of diced mango to the batter just before cooking gives these pancakes a great flavor and pleasing color.

Nutrition Facts

Per serving:

220 calories

7g protein

36g carbohydrates

7g fat

Oven-dried persimmon rounds

Ingredients

• 6 medium fuyu persimmons

Preparation

• Preheat oven to 250F.

• Thinly slice the persimmons crosswise into 1/4-inch rounds.

• Divide the persimmons between 2 wire racks set atop baking sheets.

• Bake until the centers look dry and the edges begin to curl up, about 1 1/2 to 2 hours.

• Store in an airtight container in the refrigerator.

Grilled chicken salad with greens

• 4 servings

• Ingredients: Ingredient Checklist

• 4 (6-ounce) skinless, boneless chicken breast halves

• 1 tablespoon olive oil

- ½ teaspoon salt

- ½ teaspoon freshly ground black pepper

- Cooking spray

- ⅓ cup finely chopped celery

- ⅓ cup sweetened dried cranberries

- ¼ cup chopped pecans, toasted

- 3 tablespoons light sour cream

- 3 tablespoons canola mayonnaise

- 2 teaspoons fresh lemon juice

Directions: Instructions Checklist

Step 1

- Preheat grill to medium-high heat.

Step 2

- Brush both sides of chicken evenly with oil; sprinkle with salt and pepper. Place chicken on a grill rack coated with cooking spray; grill 6 minutes on each side or until done. Let stand 10 minutes; shred. Place chicken in a large bowl. Add celery and next 3 ingredients; toss.

Step 3

- Combine sour cream and remaining ingredients, stirring well. Add sour cream mixture to chicken mixture; toss to coat.

• Serve this main-dish salad over fresh spinach. Regular spinach is the least expensive option, but you'll have to remove the stems. If time is your main concern, buy baby spinach.

Nutrition Facts

• Per Serving: 391 calories; fat 22g; saturated fat 3.4g; mono fat 11.4g; poly fat 5.1g; protein 36.1g; carbohydrates 11.5g; fiber 1.8g; cholesterol 101mg; iron 1.6mg; sodium 469mg; calcium 59mg.

Scramled egg with spinach
Yield: Serves 1

Ingredients: Ingredient Checklist

• 1 teaspoon unsalted butter

• 2 large eggs

• ¼ teaspoon freshly ground black pepper

• ⅛ teaspoon kosher salt

Directions

Step 1

• Melt your butter in an 8-inch nonstick skillet over medium-high until it gets bubbly; diner-style scrambles do not fear heat.

Step 2

• While butter melts, break eggs into a small bowl. Use a fork to beat them like they owe you money until completely blended and slightly frothy. Stir in the pepper and salt.

Step 3

• Add egg mixture to pan; start pulling the eggs from the sides of the pan into the middle (the edges cook faster than the center). Big, fluffy curds will start to form-- exactly what you want. Keep it up, pulling the eggs from around the pan for about 3 minutes. The second all the runny egg is fully set--there's an eggshell-thin line between fluffy, firm eggs and tough, dry ones--pull the pan from the heat and slide the eggs onto your plate.

• Serve this scrambled egg over fresh spinach

Nutrition Facts

• Per Serving: 179 calories; fat 13.4g; saturated fat 5.6g; mono fat 4.7g; poly fat 2.1g; protein 13g; carbohydrates 1g; cholesterol 382mg; iron 2mg; sodium 383mg; calcium 59mg.

oven-dried persimmon rounds
Ingredients:

- 1 pound ground turkey

- ½ cup panko

- ¼ cup finely chopped cilantro

- 1 tablespoon finely chopped fresh ginger

- 3 scallions, white and light-green parts, chopped

- 2 cloves garlic, minced

- 1 large egg

- 3 tablespoons low-sodium soy sauce

- ¼ cup hoisin sauce

- ¼ cup plum sauce

- 1 tablespoon rice vinegar

- Rice or rice noodles, optional

Directions:

Step 1

Combine turkey, panko, cilantro, ginger, scallions, garlic, egg and 1 Tbsp. soy sauce. Mix gently with your hands (do not overmix), then form into 16 balls. Place in slow cooker.

Step 2

Combine remaining 2 Tbsp. soy sauce, hoisin sauce, plum sauce and rice vinegar. Pour over meatballs. Cover and cook on low until meatballs are cooked through, 2 1/2 to 3 hours. Serve over rice or with noodles, if desired.

Cooking and Serving Tips

Need a more calorie dense snack? Quarter these persimmon rounds and use them in a homemade trailmix. Try mixing them with walnuts, pumpkin seeds, and dark chocolate chips. You can also add them to a cup of Greek yogurt for a protein and calcium-rich snack.

Include these oven-dried persimmon rounds in your favorite salad for an extra crunch of fiber, Vitamin C, and antioxidants.2

This is a great recipe to have leftovers from because it is so versatile. Make a large batch for the whole week and have them morning, afternoon, or evening to satisfy a sweet, crunchy craving. They are a unique Thanksgiving addition to your appetizer or dessert platter. Pour them in a lined basket and enjoy a festive fall snack. Or, pair them with a batch of kale chips for an extra crunchy and nutrient-rich snack.

Banana Breakfast Smoothie

Yield: 2 servings (serving size: 1 cup)

This protein-packed smoothie is perfect for breakfast on the go. Adding the yogurt at the very end imparts a creamy texture.

Ingredients:

• ½ cu½ cup 1% low-fat milk

• p crushed ice

• 1 tablespoon honey

• ⅛ teaspoon ground nutmeg

• 1 frozen sliced ripe large banana

• 1 cup plain 2% reduced-fat Greek yogurt

Directions: Step 1

• Combine first 5 ingredients in a blender; process 2 minutes or until smooth. Add yogurt; process just until blended. Serve immediately.

Baked chicken with cauliflower rice
4 servings

Ingredients

• 1 head cauliflower, broken into florets

• 1 tablespoon butter

• 1 tablespoon olive oil

• 2 tablespoons minced fresh parsley

• 1 tablespoon minced garlic, or more to taste

• 1 teaspoon poultry seasoning

• 2 cups shredded cooked chicken

• 1 (10.75 ounce) can condensed cream of mushroom soup

• ½ cup mozzarella cheese

• ½ cup whole milk

• salt to taste

• 1 large bell peppers, stemmed and seeded

Directions

• Preheat oven to 400 degrees F (200 degrees C).

• Place cauliflower florets in a food processor; pulse into rice-sized pieces.

• Heat butter and oil in a large skillet over medium heat.; cook and stir for 2 minutes. Add cauliflower "rice"; cook, stirring frequently, until softened, about 5 minutes. Stir in parsley, garlic, and poultry seasoning. Cook until fragrant, about 1 minute. Remove from heat.

• Stir chicken, mozzarella cheese, milk, salt, and pepper into the "rice" mixture.

• Season chicken and stuffed with the bell pepper. Cover baking dish with aluminum foil.

• Bake in the preheated oven until heated through, about 30 minutes. Uncover and continue baking until golden brown, about 15 minutes more.

Notes:

• Coarsely grate cauliflower with a hand grater instead of a food processor if preferred.

• Substitute half-and-half for the milk if desired.

• Substitute ground sage for the poultry seasoning if desired.

Nutrition Facts (per serving)

405 Calories

20g Fat

29g Carbs

31g Protein

Whole grain pancakes with blueberries

Ingredients

Yield: About 10 pancakes

• 1cup whole-wheat flour

• ¾cup all-purpose flour

• ½cup cornmeal

• ¼cup rolled oats

• 2teaspoons baking powder

• 1teaspoon kosher salt

- ½teaspoon baking soda

- 2¼cups buttermilk or plain yogurt (not Greek)

- 3large eggs

- ½ cup fresh blueberries

- ¼cup unsalted butter, melted, plus more for serving

- 1tablespoon honey

- Maple syrup, for serving

Preparation

Step 1

In a large bowl, mix together whole-wheat flour, all-purpose flour, cornmeal, oats, baking powder, salt and baking soda. In a medium bowl, mix together buttermilk, eggs, melted butter and honey. Mix the egg mixture into the flour mixture until smooth.

Step 2

Heat a griddle or large cast-iron skillet over medium heat. Check to see if it's hot by sprinkling a few drops of water on the surface. They should sizzle and evaporate immediately.

Step 3

Add a little butter to the pan and let it melt. Pour about ⅓ cup batter onto skillet; Sprinkle a few blueberries into the wet batter. Cook until pancakes are evenly browned,

3 to 4 minutes per side. Repeat with remaining batter and blueberries, leaving space for each pancake to spread.

Step 4

Cook until bubbles form and start to burst, about 3 minutes. Flip and cook until golden on the other side, 2 to 3 minutes. Transfer to a plate as they finish, and serve immediately with maple syrup and more butter on top, if you like.

Step 5

Repeat with the remaining batter, adding more butter to the skillet as needed.

Blueberry Chia Pudding

Ingredients

• Almond milk: Start with two cups of almond milk. You can use oat milk, coconut milk, or cow's milk if you prefer.

• Chia seeds: Chia seeds are a great source of fiber, antioxidants, and omega-3 fatty acids.

• Blueberries: Choose firm blueberries that are fragrant and deeply colored. Avoid berries that are bruised or wrinkled.

• Maple syrup and vanilla: Maple syrup and vanilla extract lend sweetness and complex flavor.

• Cinnamon: Take the flavor up a notch with a pinch of ground cinnamon.

Direction

Combine the ingredients in a blender, blend until smooth, and pour into ramekins or glasses. Chill until set (8 hours to overnight) and serve. That's all there is to it!

Steak with roated veggies

Yield: 4 people

Ingredients

veggies

• 2 zucchini, sliced into half-circles

• 2 yellow squash, sliced into half-circles

• ½ pint grape or small cherry tomatoes

• 3 tbsp olive or avocado oil

• ½ tsp garlic powder

• ½ tsp dried oregano

• ½ tsp salt

Steak

• 1 lb sirloin steak, thinly sliced, about ½-inch thick pieces

• 2 tbsp coconut aminos or soy sauce

- ½ tsp salt

- ½ tsp pepper

- ¼ tsp crushed red pepper flakes

- ¼ tsp garlic powder

Instruction

- Preheat the oven to 425°F. Line a 12" x 17" baking sheet with parchment paper.

- Combine steak with coconut aminos, salt, pepper, crushed red pepper flakes, and garlic powder. Set aside. (While you can marinate for up to 12 hours, there is no need with this recipe. Just let it sit in the marinade ingredients while your veggies are roasting and you'll be good to go!)

- Spread zucchini, and squash on the baking sheet. They do not need to be kept separate. Drizzle with olive oil. Sprinkle with garlic powder, dried oregano, and salt. Stir so everything is well seasoned. Spread in a single layer after stirring.

- Place in the oven and bake for 20 minutes or until veggies are softened and close to done.

- Spread marinated steak on baking sheet with veggies. Bake for 5 to 8 minutes, or until steak is how you like it.

Nutritional fact

calories: 311kcal, carbohydrates: 14g, protein: 28g, fat: 16g, saturated fat: 4g, cholesterol: 69mg, sodium: 836mg, potassium: 1069mg, fiber: 3g, sugar: 7g, vitamin a: 718iu, vitamin c: 50mg, calcium: 79mg, iron: 3mg

How long should you marinate the steak?

You can marinate your steak for up to 12 hours. For this recipe I just let the marinade work it's magic in the 20 minutes I have while the veggies are roasting. There isn't much liquid to this marinade and it's designed to work quickly!

Tuna Salad with Cranberries

This simple, unusual cranberry tuna salad recipe will yield the best sandwiches you've ever had! Try on potato bread for a comforting, yummy treat!

Ingredients

Directions

Place tuna in a bowl, and mash with a fork. Mix in mayonnaise to evenly coat tuna. Mix in dill and cranberries, and season with salt. Enjoy on crackers or the bread of your choice!

Nutrition Facts (per serving)

140 Calories

6g Fat

5g Carbs

16g Protein

Cottage Cheese Chicken Enchiladas

Ever tried chicken enchiladas made with cottage cheese?
Now's your chance! This takes some prep time, but it is
well worth it. You can make it 1 day ahead, and serve
the next day.

Yield:6 servings

Ingredients

• 1 tablespoon vegetable oil

• 2 skinless, boneless chicken breast halves - boiled and
shredded

• ½ cup chopped onion

• 1 (7 ounce) can chopped green chile peppers

• 1 (1 ounce) package taco seasoning mix

• ½ cup sour cream

• 2 cups cottage cheese

• 1 teaspoon salt

• 1 pinch ground black pepper

• 12 (6 inch) corn tortillas

• 2 cups shredded Monterey Jack cheese

• 1 (10 ounce) can red enchilada sauce

Directions

• To Make Meat Mixture: Heat oil in medium skillet over medium high heat. Add chicken, onion and green chile peppers and saute until browned, then add taco seasoning and prepare meat mixture according to package directions.

• To Make Cheese Mixture: In a medium bowl mix sour cream with cottage cheese and season with salt and pepper; stir until well blended.

• Preheat oven to 350 degrees F (175 degrees C).

• To Assemble Enchiladas: Heat tortillas until soft. In each tortilla place a spoonful of meat mixture, a spoonful of cheese mixture and a bit of shredded cheese. Roll tortillas and place in a lightly greased 9x13 inch baking dish. Top with any remaining meat and cheese mixture, enchilada sauce and remaining shredded cheese.

• Bake at 350 degrees F (175 degrees C) for 30 minutes or until cheese is melted and bubbly.

Nutrition Facts (per serving)

549 Calories

31g Fat

34g Carbs

33g Protein

Cinnamon-Peach Cottage Cheese Pancakes

A cottage cheese-based pancake with fruit for extra flavor.

Servings:4

Yield:12 pancakes

Ingredients

• 4 eggs

• 1 cup cottage cheese

• ½ cup milk

• 1 teaspoon vanilla extract

• 2 tablespoons butter, melted

• 1 peach, shredded

• 1 cup all-purpose flour

• 2 tablespoons white sugar

• 1 pinch salt

• ¾ teaspoon baking soda

• 1 teaspoon ground cinnamon

Directions

• Mix eggs, cottage cheese, milk, vanilla, butter, and peach in a large bowl. Combine flour, sugar, salt, baking soda, and cinnamon in a small bowl. Stir flour mixture into the cottage cheese mixture until just combined.

• Heat a lightly oiled griddle over medium-high heat. Drop batter by large spoonful onto the griddle, and cook until bubbles form and the edges are dry. Flip, and cook until browned on the other side. Repeat with remaining batter.

Nutrition Facts (per serving)

• 344 Calories

• 14g Fat

• 36g Carbs

• 18g Protein

Cinnamon-Curry Tuna Salad

Yield: 4 servings

Ingredients

• 2 (5 ounce) cans water packed tuna, drained and flaked

• 2 teaspoons mayonnaise

• 1 teaspoon Dijon mustard

• 1 tablespoon sweet pickle relish

• 2 teaspoons lemon juice

• 1 ½ teaspoons ground cinnamon

• 1 teaspoon curry powder

• 1 teaspoon ground black pepper

• salt to taste

Directions

In a bowl, mix the tuna, mayonnaise, mustard, relish, lemon juice, cinnamon, curry powder, pepper, and salt. Cover, and refrigerate until ready to serve.

Nutrition Facts (per serving)

102 Calories

3g Fat

3g Carbs

16g Protein

Apple almond pie

Recipe Summary

This is the sweet lover's apple pie. Surprising ingredients make this apple pie stand out from the rest!

Prep:30 mins

Cook:45 mins

Total:1 hr 15 mins

Servings:8

Yield:1- 9 inch pie

Ingredients

- 1 (15 ounce) package pastry for a double crust 9-inch pie, divided

- 6 cups peeled and sliced apples

- ½ cup crushed almonds

- 1 ¼ cups white sugar

- ½ cup brown sugar

- 2 tablespoons all-purpose flour

- 2 tablespoons honey

- 1 large egg yolk

- ½ teaspoon water

- ¼ teaspoon almond extract

- 1 teaspoon ground cinnamon, or to taste

Directions

Step 1

Preheat oven to 350 degrees F (175 degrees C). Press 1 pie crust into a 9-inch pie pan.

Step 2

Toss apples, almonds, white sugar, brown sugar, and flour together in a bowl until apples and almonds are completely coated.

Step 3

Mix honey, egg yolk, water, and almond extract together in a microwave-safe dish.

 Step 4

Microwave honey mixture, stirring every 15 seconds, until mixture is melted and smooth, 30 to 45 seconds. Pour honey mixture over apple mixture and toss to coat. Transfer apple mixture to the prepared pie crust; sprinkle filling with cinnamon. Top pie with the remaining pie crust and pinch edges together to seal.

 Step 5

Bake in the preheated oven until crust is lightly browned, 45 to 50 minutes.

Nutrition Facts

Per Serving: 533 calories; protein 5.1g; carbohydrates 87.2g; fat 19.9g; cholesterol 25.6mg; sodium 259.2mg.

Caramel Apple Crumble Pie

So delicious and sweet! This pie, with its pastry crust and cinnamon-spiced oat topping, is the perfect combination of caramel apple pie and apple crumble.

Servings: 8

Yield: 1 to 9 - inch pie

Ingredients

FOR THE CRUMBLE TOPPING

- 1 cup rolled oats

- ½ cup brown sugar

- ¼ cup all-purpose flour

- ½ cup slivered almonds

- ¼ teaspoon ground cinnamon

- ¼ cup butter, cubed

FOR THE PIE

- 1 (9 inch) single pie crust

- 6 apples - peeled, cored, and thinly sliced

- 2 tablespoons lemon juice

- 1 tablespoon all-purpose flour

- ½ cup brown sugar

- 2 teaspoons ground cinnamon

- ½ cup caramel sauce

Preheat an oven to 350 degrees F (175 degrees C).

To make the topping, combine the oats, 1/2 cup brown sugar, 1/4 cup flour, slivered almonds, and 1/4 teaspoon cinnamon. Cut in the butter until the mixture resembles coarse crumbs; set aside.

Roll out the pie dough into a circle and transfer it to a 9-inch pie plate. Trim the pastry and crimp the edge. Toss the apples with the lemon juice in a bowl to prevent browning. Combine the 1 tablespoon flour, 1/2 cup brown sugar, and 2 teaspoons cinnamon; toss with the apples to coat. Drizzle 1/4 cup of caramel sauce over the bottom of the pie shell. Add the spiced apple mixture; drizzle with remaining 1/4 cup of caramel sauce. Sprinkle the crumble topping evenly over the apples.

Bake the pie in the preheated oven for 50-60 minutes, or until the apples are tender and the crust is browned.

Nutrition Facts (per serving)

456 Calories

18g Fat

73g Carbs

5g Protein

Quinoa Vegetable Salad

This quinoa vegetable salad is a wonderful dish — it's light and very tasty. My four kids (ages 2-7) ate it up and asked for more!

Servings: 10

Yield: 5 cups

Ingredients

• 1 teaspoon canola oil

• 1 tablespoon minced garlic

- ¼ cup diced yellow (or purple) onion

- 2 ½ cups water

- 3 teaspoons salt, divided, or to taste

- 1/2 teaspoon ground black pepper, divided

- 2 cups quinoa

- ¾ cup diced fresh tomato

- ¾ cup diced carrots

- ½ cup diced yellow bell pepper

- ½ cup diced cucumber

- ½ cup frozen corn kernels, thawed

- ¼ cup diced red onion

- 1 ½ tablespoons choped fresh cilantro

- 1 tablespoon chopped fresh mint

- 3 tablespoons balsamic vinegar

- 2 tablespoons olive oil

Directions

- Heat canola oil in a saucepan over medium heat. Add garlic and yellow onion; cook and stir until onion has softened and turned translucent, about 5 minutes. Add water, 2 teaspoons salt, and 1/4 teaspoon pepper; bring to a boil.

• Stir quinoa into the pan, reduce the heat to medium-low, and cover. Simmer until quinoa is tender, about 20 minutes. Drain any remaining water with a mesh strainer; transfer quinoa to a large mixing bowl. Cover and refrigerate until cold, about 45 minutes.

• Stir tomato, carrots, bell pepper, cucumber, corn, and red onion into chilled quinoa. Season with cilantro, mint, and remaining 1 teaspoon salt and 1/4 teaspoon black pepper. Drizzle with balsamic vinegar and olive oil, then gently stir until evenly mixed.

Nutrition Facts (per serving)

99 Calories

4g Fat

14g Carbs

2g Protein

Cooking and Meal Planning

Thankfully, you won't need any special equipment or fancy tools to cook up delicious, nutritious meals on the acid reflux diet. These few tips can take you a long way:

Meal Planning and Prepping

You can save yourself a lot of time, effort, and money if you go to the grocery store with a plan in mind. Before you head out, decide what you want to eat for that week, make a list, and stick to it at the store.

After you've planned your menu and purchased your items, it's time to cook. The acid reflux diet emphasizes plenty of foods that can be prepared ahead of time and reheated on the stove or in the microwave, so you don't have to worry about meals sucking up a bunch of your time. Most vegetables, whole grains, and proteins will stay fresh in the fridge for three to five days.

Use What You Have on Hand

If you feel like you're in a pinch for ingredients, you might not actually be. The acid reflux diet isn't necessarily restrictive, so chances are you can whip up a tasty meal even when you feel like your pantry is getting bare. Think simple, like Italian-seasoned rice or rolled oats with mashed bananas.

With these LPR diet recipes, you can enjoy flavorful and nourishing meals while minimizing discomfort. By selecting the right ingredients and avoiding triggers, you can optimize your overall well-being and manage your LPR symptoms effectively

Effective and well-detailed meal plan for LPR diet

Day Breakfast Snack Lunch Snack Dinner

- Monday LPR-friendly smoothie Greek yogurt with honey Grilled chicken salad with greens Apple slices with almond butter Baked salmon with steamed broccoli
- Tuesday Scrambled egg with spinach Melon chunks Quinoa and vegetable stir-fry Carrot

sticks with hummus Turkey meatballs with zucchini noodles
- Wednesday Whole grain toast with avocado Mixed berries smoothie Tuna salad with whole grain crackers Cucumber slices with guacamole Grilled shrimp with quinoa and asparagus
- Thursday Plain yogurt with sliced peaches Rice cakes with almond butter Lentil soup with whole grain bread Sliced bell peppers with humus Grilled chicken with roasted sweet potatoes
- Friday Blueberry Chia Pudding Cottage cheese with pineapple Quinoa and black bean salad Edamame Baked cod with sautéed spinach and quinoa
- Saturday Whole grain pancakes with blueberries Trail mix Veggie wrap with salsa Sliced pear with almond butter Grilled steak with roasted vegetables
- Sunday Smoothie with kale and banana Cherry tomatoes with mozzarella Brown rice with green vegetables Mixed nuts Baked chicken with cauliflower rice

For this LPR diet, it's important to avoid acidic, spicy, and fatty foods, as well as caffeine and alcohol. The meal plan above focuses on non-acidic, low-fat, and non-spicy food choices to help manage LPR symptoms.

Conclusion

If simple, conventional LPR treatment with PPIs or H2 blockers hasn't helped you, don't despair. Making some simple changes to your diet and lifestyle and investigating your root causes may provide you with solutions that resolve your symptoms.

Focus on identifying your reflux food triggers, rebalancing your gut microbiome, supporting stomach acid if appropriate, and bringing in research-supported supplements.

The silent reflux diet is a food-based approach to reduce reflux symptoms. Though effective, these dietary changes may not treat the underlying cause of silent reflux. Traditional treatment methods shouldn't be ignored and can be used in combination with this diet.

Before incorporating the silent reflux diet into your treatment plan, discuss your options and risks with your doctor. If you begin to experience irregular symptoms, seek immediate medical attention.

The correct LPR diet is individual. You should learn to get a feeling for the right foods. Listen to your body and pay attention to which kind of foods you feel better or worse after.

Not everyone reacts in the same way to various foods. The differences depend on our genes, our way of living, and our environment. While a low-fat diet works well for most people, some people do better on a low-carb diet.

The goal of an LPR diet is not to strictly follow the rules, but to find out what works best for you. You need to figure out what tastes good and at the same time is good for you.